I0421553

# Body Scrub Recipes

## Natural Skin And Body Care Book

By : Kinjal Rambhia

Published By :

# Kinjal Rambhia

© Copyright 2015 – Kinjal Rambhia

ISBN-13: 978-1517032081
ISBN-10: 1517032083

# Table of Contents

20. Orange Body Scrub
21. Pineapple Body Scrub
22. Aloe Vera Oatmeal Scrub
23. Papaya Scrub
24. Flax Seed and Salt Scrub
25. Tomato Scrub
26. Banana Scrub

# 1 Pumpkin And Brown Sugar Scrub

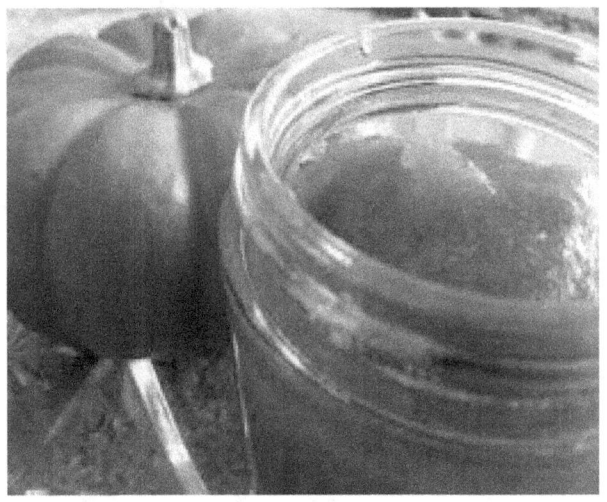

This scrub is especially for normal to dry skin.

## Ingredients

- 1 Cup Brown Sugar
- ¼ Cup Pumpkin Puree
- ½ tbsp Honey
- 1 ½ tbsp Olive Oil

## Method

- Take a bowl.

- Add pumpkin puree, olive oil and honey.
- Add brown sugar and mix it properly.
- Pour the scrub in jar and store it

## **USE**

- Remove scrub from the jar and apply it on body.
- Always scrub in circular motion for better results.
- Rinse it with warm water and apply moisturizer

# 2 Lemon Body Scrub.

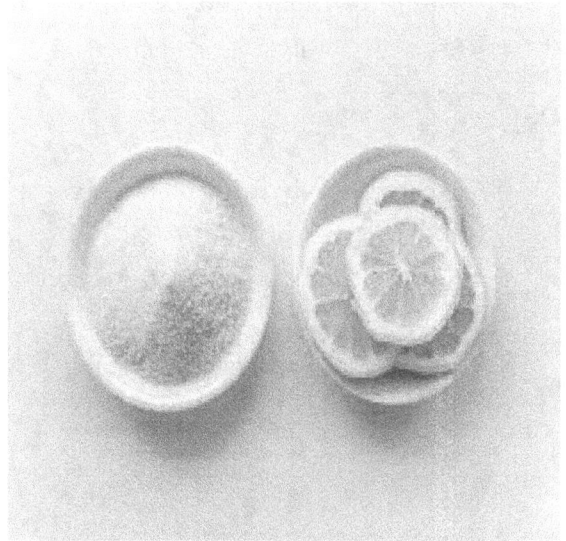

**This scrub is especially for oily and sweaty skin.**

## Ingredients

- 3 Cups of White Sugar
- ½ Cup of Olive Oil
- ½ Cup Lemon Juice
- 1 Lemon Zest
- 2 tbsp vanilla extract

## Method

- Take a bowl and add vanilla extract, olive oil, lemon juice, lemon zest and mix it evenly.
- Add White sugar in the mixture and mix it

well. Lemon scrub is ready.

## USE

- Remove scrub from the jar and apply it on body.
- Always scrub in circular motion for better results.
- Rinse it with warm water and apply moisturizer

# 3 Chocolate Body Scrub

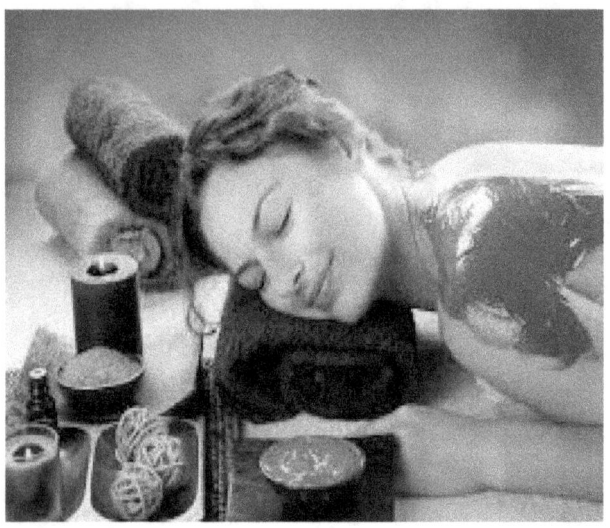

**This scrub is especially for tanned and dark skin.**

### Ingredients

- ½ Cup Coconut Oil
- ½ Cup Sweet Almond Oil
- ½ Cup Brown Sugar
- ½ Cup Coco Powder

### Method

- Combine all the ingredients in a bowl and mix it well.
- Pour in jar and store it.

### USE

- Remove scrub from the jar and apply it on body.
- Always scrub in circular motion for better results.
- Rinse it with warm water and apply moisturizer

# 4 Pepper Mint Body Scrub

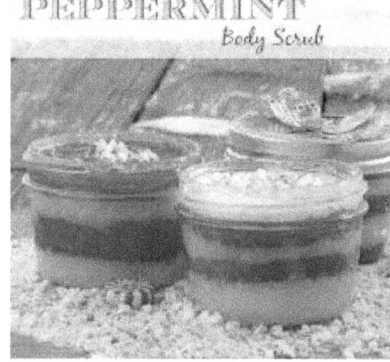
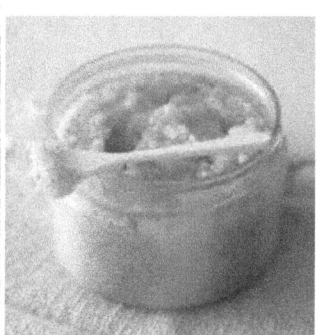

**This scrub is especially for oily and sweaty skin.**

## Ingredients

- 1 Cup Epsom Salt
- ¼ Cup  Ground Pepper.
- ½ Cup Olive Oil
- 6-8 Drops of Mint Essential Oil

## Method

- Mix all the ingredients in a bowl.
- Pour in jar and store it.

## USE

- Remove scrub from the jar and apply it on

body.

- Always scrub in circular motion for better results.
- Rinse it with warm water and apply moisturizer

# 5 Whipped Grapefruit Body Scrub

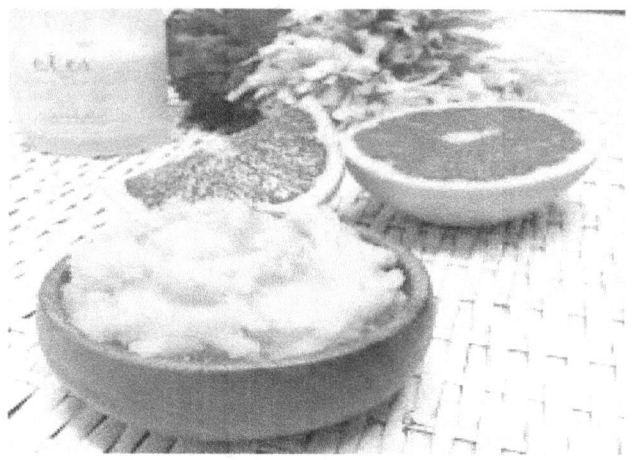

**This scrub is especially for normal to dry skin**

### Ingredients

- ½ Cup Coconut Oil
- ½ Cup White Sugar
- ½ Cup Grapefruit Zest
- 2 tbsp Grapefruit Juice
- 10 Drops Grapefruit Oil
- ¼ tbsp Beet Root Juice (For Color)

### Method

- Take firm Coconut Oil and White Sugar in a bowl and beat it with beater, until a thick foam is formed.

- Add all the remaining ingredients in the foam and beat it again.
- The mixture should be blended evenly and fluffy foam should be created.
- Store in an air-tight jar in the refrigerator.

## USE

- Remove scrub from the jar and apply it on body.
- Always scrub in circular motion for better results.
- Rinse it with warm water and apply moisturizer

# 6 Banana Moisturizing Body Scrub

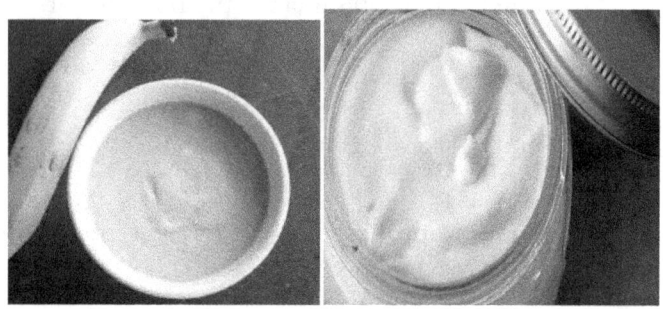

This scrub is especially for normal to dry and excessive dry skin.

Even sensitive skin can use this scrub.

<u>Ingredients</u>

- ¼ Cup Shea Butter
- ¼ Cup Coconut Butter
- ¼ Cup Almond Oil
- ¼ Apricot Kernel Oil
- 1 Ripe Banana
- 1 Cup White Sugar

<u>Method</u>

- In a blender pour Shea butter, coconut butter, almond oil, apricot kernel oil, and banana.

- Blend it until it becomes fine paste.
- Take a jar, add sugar and pour the blended paste in it.
- Stir sugar properly in the paste.
- Store in air-tight jar in the refrigerator.

## USE

- Remove scrub from the jar and apply it on body.
- Always scrub in circular motion for better results.
- Rinse it with warm water and apply moisturizer

# 7 Mango Body Scrub

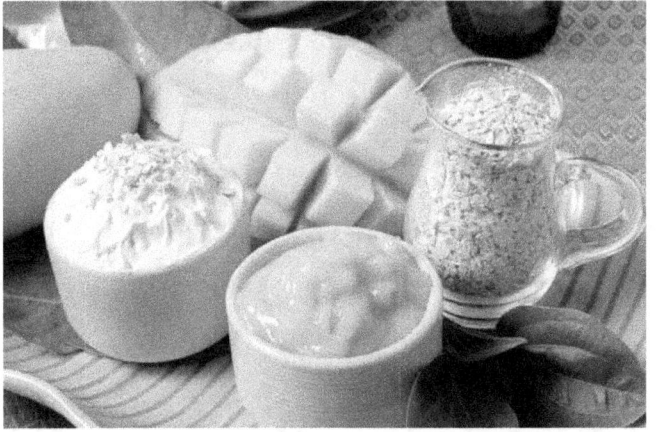

## This scrub will give you de-tanning effect.

### Ingredients

- ¼ Cup Fresh Mango Puree.
- ½ Cup Oats
- 1 tbsp Coconut Oil
- 1 tbsp Orange Juice

### Method

- Mix all the ingredients in a bowl.
- Pour in jar and store it.

### USE

- Store in the refrigerator
- Remove scrub from the jar and apply it on body.

- Always scrub in circular motion for better results.
- Rinse it with warm water and apply moisturizer

# 8 Vanilla Sugar Body Scrub

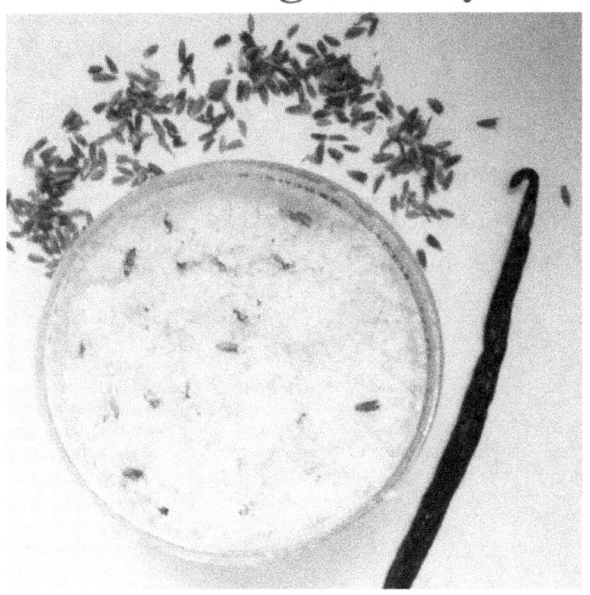

**This scrub is recommended for sensitive skin**

## Ingredients

- 1 Cup Fine Brown Sugar
- 1/3 Cup Base Oil (your choice of oil almond, olive, argon oil etc)
- 1 tbsp Vanilla Essence

## Method

- Mix all the ingredients in a bowl.
- Pour in jar and store it.

## USE

- Remove scrub from the jar and apply it on body.
- Always scrub in circular motion for better results.
- Rinse it with warm water and apply moisturizer

# 9 Oatmeal Body Scrub

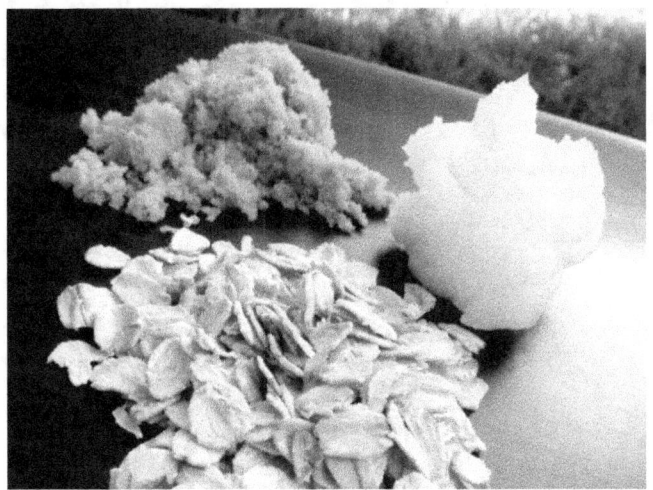

**This scrub is for all skin type.**

## Ingredients

- 1 Cup finely ground Oats
- 2 tbsp dried Lavender Petals
- 10 Drops Lavender essential oil
- 6 Drops Chamomile

## Method

- Mix all the ingredients in a bowl.
- Pour in jar and store it.

## USE

- Remove scrub from the jar and apply it on body.

- Always scrub in circular motion for better results.
- Rinse it with warm water and apply moisturizer

# 10 Honey And Oats Body Scrub

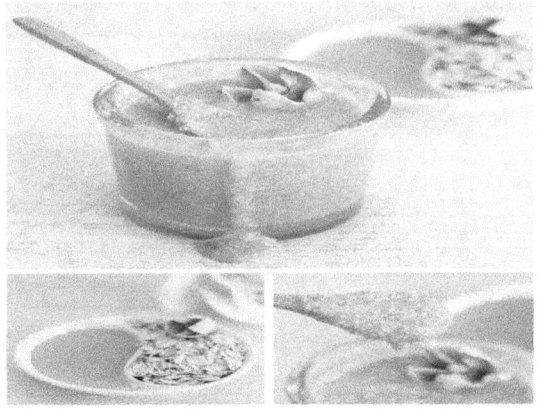

**This scrub is for all skin type.**

## Ingredients

- ½ Cup finely ground Oats
- 2 tbsp Honey
- 2 tbsp Olive Oil
- 2-3 tbsp Milk

## Method

- Mix all the ingredients in a bowl.
- Pour in jar and store it.

## USE

- Remove scrub from the jar and apply it on body.

- Always scrub in circular motion for better results.
- Rinse it with warm water and apply moisturizer

# 11 Rosemary Salt Scrub

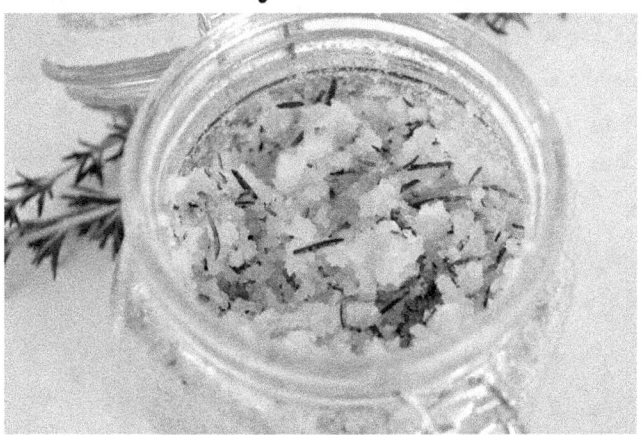

**This scrub is recommended for dry and dull skin.**

## Ingredients

- 1 Cup Salt
- 1/3 Cup Sweet Almond Oil
- ½ Cup Dried Rosemary leaves
- 6-8 Drops Rosemary essential Oil

## Method

- Mix all the ingredients in a bowl.
- Pour in jar and store it.

## USE

- Remove scrub from the jar and apply it on

body.

- Always scrub in circular motion for better results.
- Rinse it with warm water and apply moisturizer

# 12 Latte Sugar Scrub

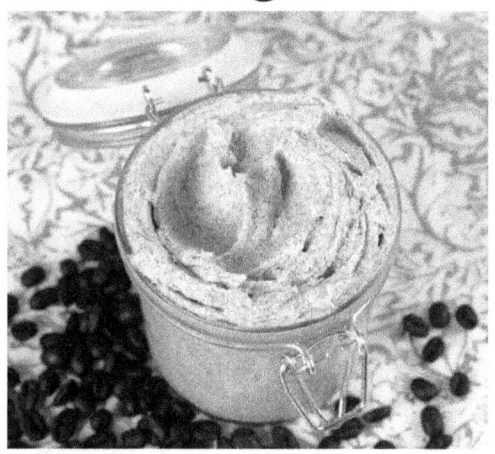

**This scrub is recommended for dry and dull skin.**

## Ingredients

- ½ Cup finely ground coffee
- ½ Cup organic Sugar
- 2 tbsp coconut oil
- 2 tbsp Castor oil

## Method

- Mix all the ingredients in a bowl.
- Pour in jar and store it.

## USE

- Remove scrub from the jar and apply it on body.

- Always scrub in circular motion for better results.
- Rinse it with warm water and apply moisturizer

# 13 All Spice Body Scrub

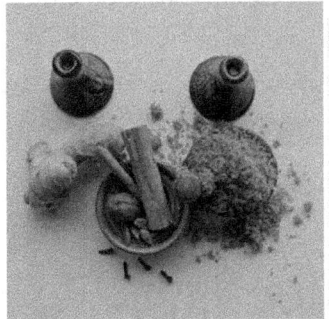 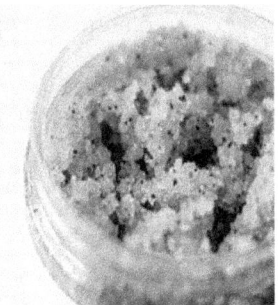

**This scrub is recommended for all skin type**

## Ingredients

- 1 Cup Sugar
- ½ Cup Carrier Oil (any oil)
- ¼ Cup Almond oil
- ½ tbsp vanilla extract
- ½ tbsp cinnamon powder
- ½ tbsp all spice powder
- ¼ tbsp Ginger

## Method

- Mix all the ingredients in a bowl.
- Pour in jar and store it.

## USE

- Remove scrub from the jar and apply it on

body.

- Always scrub in circular motion for better result.
- Rinse it with warm water and apply moisturizer

# 14 Rose Honey Scrub

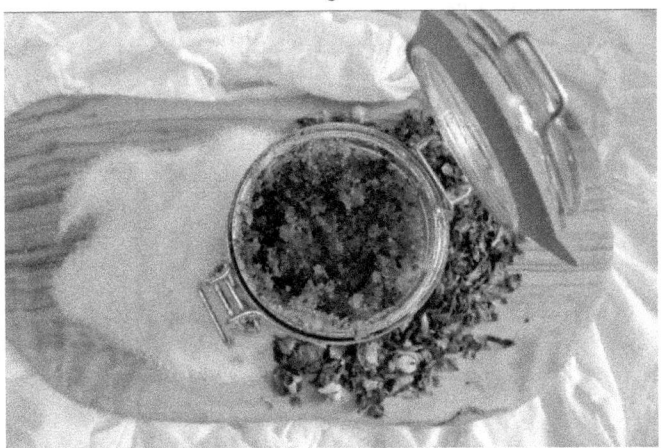

This scrub is recommended for all skin type.

## Ingredients

- 1 Cup organic sugar
- ¼ Cup Olive Oil
- 2 tbsp Raw Honey
- 3 tbsp Dried Rose petals
- 15 Drops Rose Essence
- 15 Drops Lavender Essence

## Method

- Mix all the ingredients in a bowl.
- Pour in jar and store it.

## USE

- Remove scrub from the jar and apply it on body.
- Always scrub in circular motion for better results.
- Rinse it with warm water and apply moisturizer

# 15 Vanilla Coffee Sugar Scrub Cubes

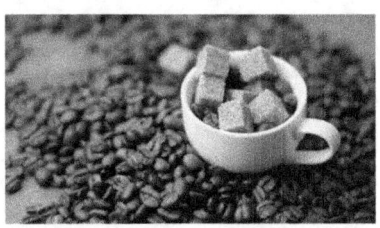

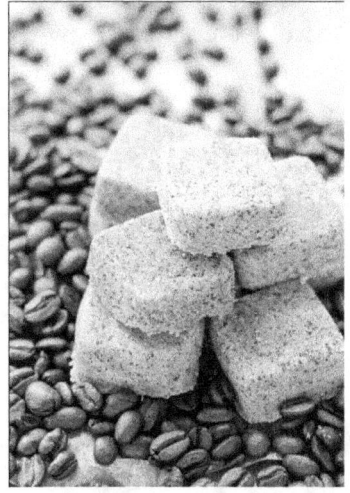

**Specially use to reduce cellulite.**

## Ingredients

- ¼ Cup Vanilla Extract
- ½ Cup Ground Coffee
- ½ Cup unscented Soap, shredded

## Method

- Take double boiler and melt the soap.

- Once the soap is melted and becomes liquid add all the ingredients.
- Mix evenly and pour into silicon molds or ice tray.
- Allow to set for minimum 3-4 hours before unmolding.

## <u>USE</u>

- You can use this scrub alternate day while bath.
- Do not use regularly as this will be too harsh for skin and will sensitized the skin.
- Rinse it with warm water and apply moisturizer
- moisturizer

# 16 Maple Sugar Scrub Cubes

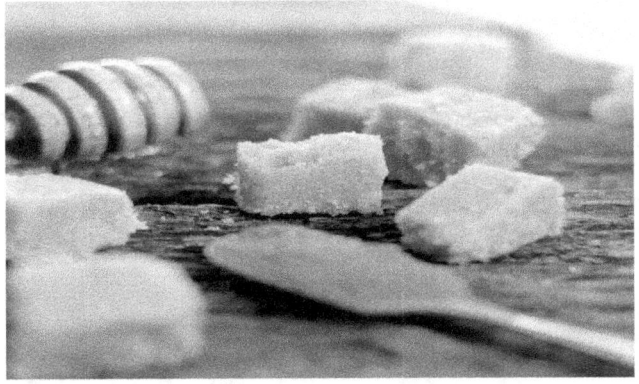

**This scrub is recommended for all skin type.**

## Ingredients

- ¼ Cup Maple extract
- 1 Cup Brown Sugar
- 6 Drops Lavender Essential Oil
- ½ Cup unscented Soap, shredded

## Method

- Take double boiler and melt the soap.
- Once the soap is melted and becomes liquid add all the ingredients.
- Mix evenly and pour into silicon molds or ice tray.
- Allow to set for minimum 3-4 hours before unmolding.

## USE

- You can use this scrub alternate day while bath.
- Do not use regularly as this will be too harsh for skin and will sensitized the skin.
- Rinse it with warm water and apply moisturizer

# 17 Almond And Sugar Scrub

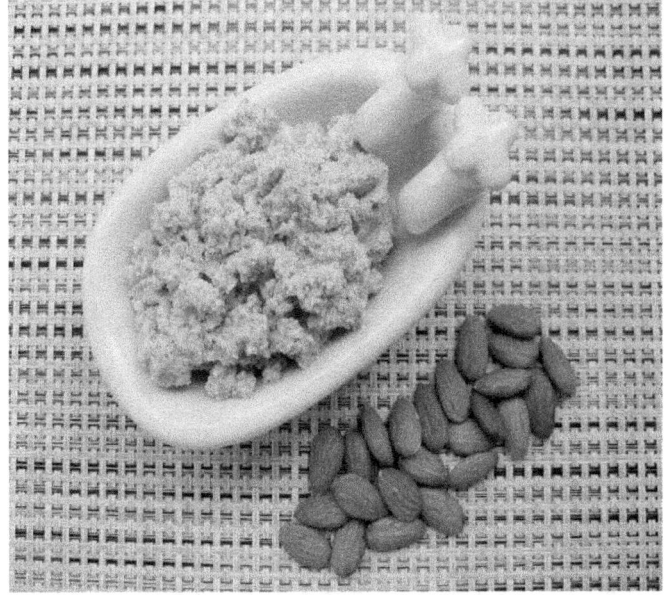

This scrub is recommended for normal to dry skin.

## Ingredients

- ¼ Cup Almond Flour
- ¼ Cup Brown Sugar
- 2 tbsp Almond oil
- 2tbsp Honey

## Method

- Mix all the ingredients in a bowl.
- Pour in jar and store it.

# USE

- Remove scrub from the jar and apply it on body.
- Always scrub in circular motion for better results
- Rinse it with warm water and apply moisturizer

# 18 Strawberry Scrub

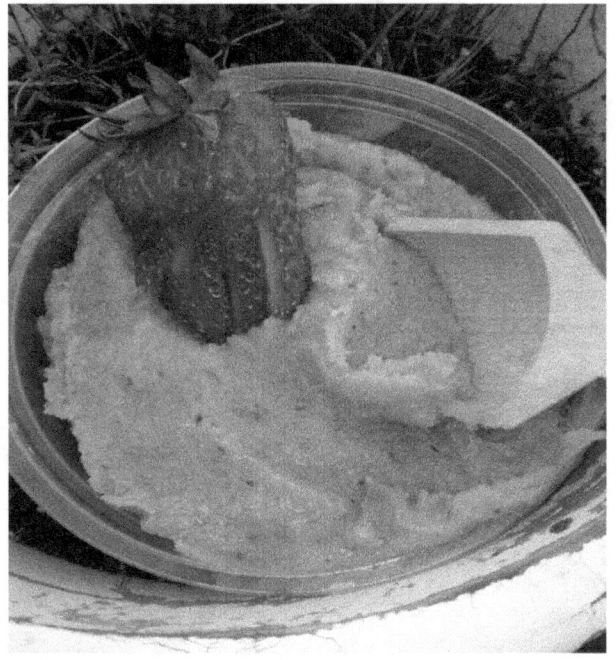

This scrub is recommended for all skin type.

## Ingredients

- ¼ Cup fresh Strawberry Crush
- ½ Cup Oats
- 1tbsp Honey

## Method

- Mix all the ingredients in a bowl.
- Pour in jar and store it.

## USE

- Remove scrub from the jar and apply it on body.
- Always scrub in circular motion for better results
- Rinse it with warm water and apply moisturizer

# 19 Coconut Body Scrub

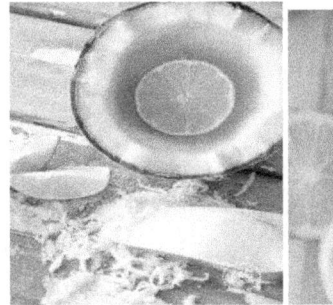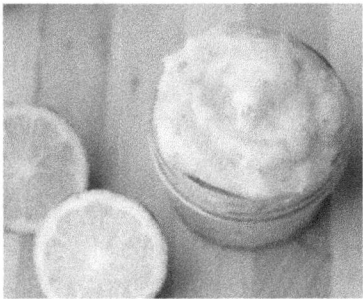

**This scrub is recommended for normal to dry and dull skin.**

## Ingredients

- ½ Cup desiccated Coconut
- ¼ Cup Coconut Oil
- 8-12 Drops Lime Essential Oil
- 4tbsp White Sugar

## Method

- Mix all the ingredients in a bowl.
- Pour in jar and store it.

## USE

- Remove scrub from the jar and apply it on body.
- Always scrub in circular motion for better

results

- Rinse it with warm water and apply moisturizer

# 20 Orange Body Scrub

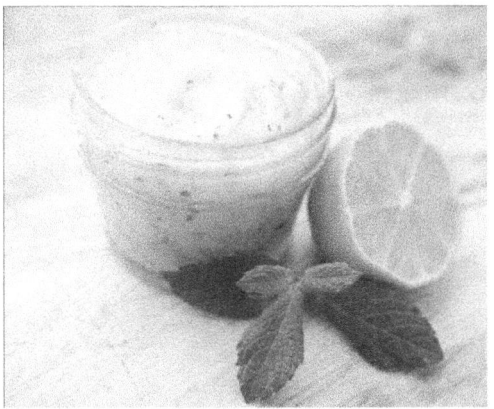

**This scrub is recommended for oily and greasy skin.**

## Ingredients

- ¼ Cup Orange Powder (dried orange skin powder)
- 3 tbsp Orange Juice
- 3tbsp Sea Salt
- 1tbsp Honey

## Method

- Mix all the ingredients in a bowl.
- Pour in jar and store it.

## USE

- Remove scrub from the jar and apply it on body.

- Always scrub in circular motion for better results
- Rinse it with warm water and apply moisturizer

# 21 Pineapple Body Scrub

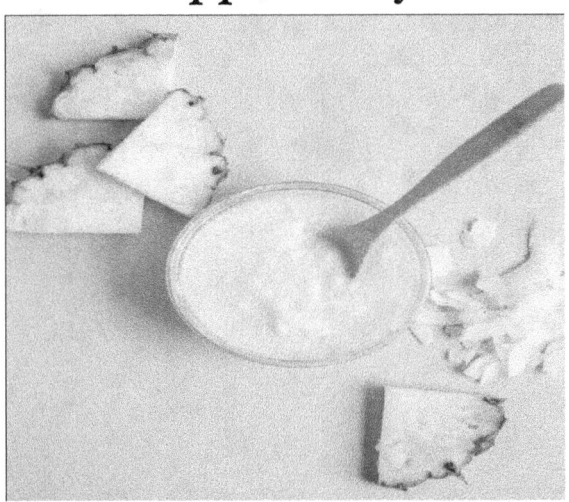

**This scrub is recommended especially for tanned and dull skin.**

## Ingredients

- ½ Cup Rice flour
- ¼ Cup Fresh Pineapple Juice

## Method

- Take rice flour in a small bowl and add fresh pineapple juice.
- Make fine paste.

## USE

- Apply paste on body and keep it for 10 minutes.

- Wet hands and scrub in circular movements.
- Rinse it with warm water and apply moisturizer

# 22 Aloe Vera Oatmeal Scrub

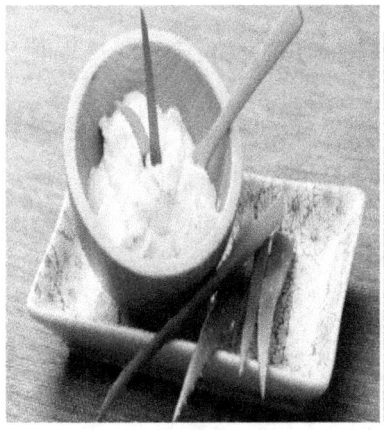 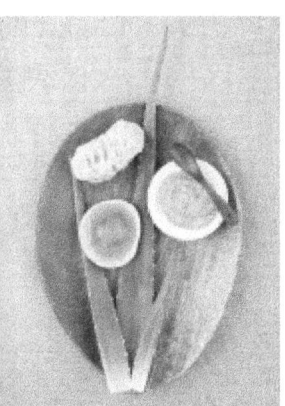

This scrub will give you hydration and nourishment to the skin.

## Ingredients

- ¼ Cup raw Oatmeal
- 2 tbsp Aloe Vera Gel
- 1 tbsp Olive Oil
- 2 tbsp Honey

## Method

- Mix all the ingredients in a bowl.
- Pour in jar and store it.

## USE

- Remove scrub from the jar and apply it on body.

- Always scrub in circular motion for better results
- Rinse it with warm water and apply moisturizer

# 23 Papaya Scrub

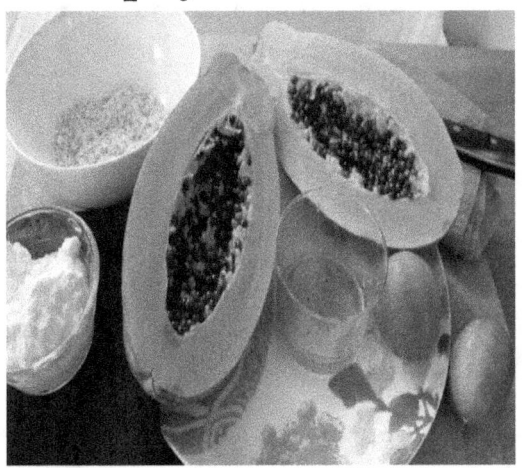

**This scrub is recommended for tanning and pigmentation**

## Ingredients

- ¼ Cup mash Papaya
- 2 tbsp yogurt
- 4 Drops Rosemary Oil
- 2 tbsp Honey

## Method

- Mix all the ingredients in a bowl.
- Pour in jar and store it.

## USE

- Remove scrub from the jar and apply it on

body.

- Always scrub in circular motion for better results
- Rinse it with warm water and apply moisturizer

# 24 Flax Seed And Salt Scrub

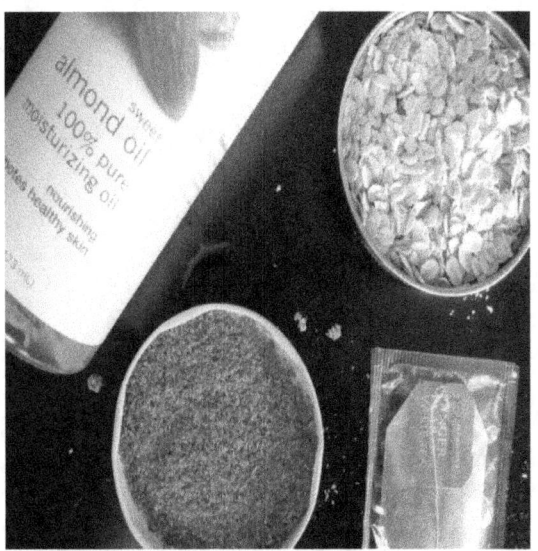

This scrub is recommended for all skin type.

## Ingredients

- 1 Cup Sea Salt
- ¼ Cup Raw Oatmeal
- 8tbsp Flax Seed Oil
- 1tbsp Olive Oil
- 8 Drops Geranium Oil

## Method

- Mix all the ingredients in a bowl.
- Pour in jar and store it.

## <u>USE</u>

- Remove scrub from the jar and apply it on body.
- Always scrub in circular motion for better results
- Rinse it with warm water and apply moisturizer

# 25 Tomato Scrub

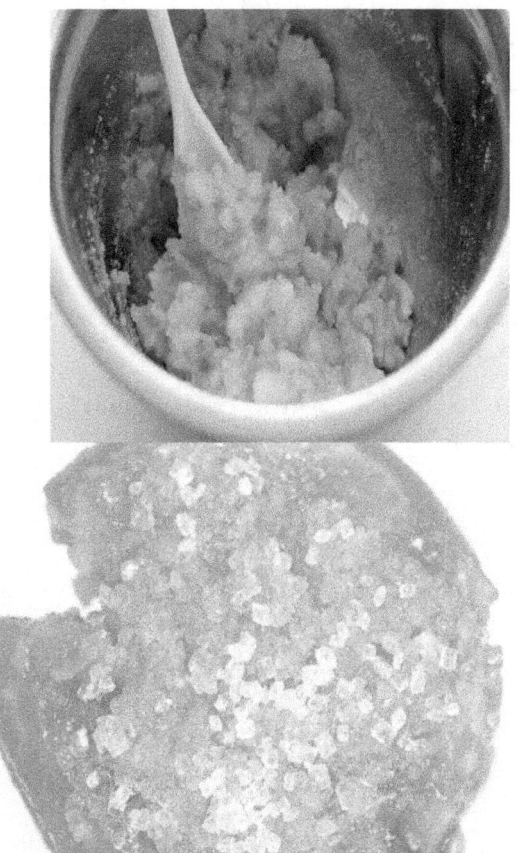

**This scrub is recommended for whitening**

## Ingredients

- ½ Cup Fresh Tomato puree
- ½ Cup Oats
- 4tbsp Sugar
- 2 tbsp Olive Oil

## Method

- Mix all the ingredients in a bowl.
- Pour in jar and store it.

## USE

- Remove scrub from the jar and apply it on body.
- Always scrub in circular motion for better results
- Rinse it with warm water and apply moisturizer

# 26 Banana Scrub

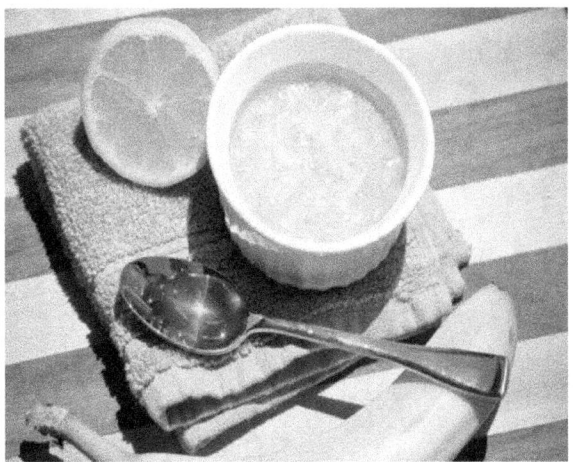

**This scrub is recommended for normal to dry skin.**

## Ingredients

- 2 mash Banana
- 5tbsp White Sugar
- 1tbsp Honey

## Method

- Mix all the ingredients in a bowl.
- Pour in jar and store it.

## USE

- Remove scrub from the jar and apply it on body.

- Always scrub in circular motion for better results
- Rinse it with warm water and apply moisturizer

## DISCLAIMER AND/OR LEGAL NOTICES:

Every effort has been made to accurately represent this book and it's potential. Results vary with every individual, and your results may or may not be different from those depicted. No promises, guarantees or warranties, whether stated or implied, have been made that you will produce any specific result from this book. Your efforts are individual and unique, and may vary from those shown. Your success depends on your efforts, background and motivation.

The material in this publication is provided for educational and informational purposes only and is not intended as medical advice. The information contained in this book should not be used to diagnose or treat any illness, metabolic disorder, disease or health problem. Always consult your physician or health care provider before beginning any nutrition or exercise program. Use of the programs, advice, and information contained in this book is at the sole choice and risk of the reader.